Meaningful Moves

Optimize Your Baby's Development

DR. SARAH E. LANE

NEWMAN SPRINGS PUBLISHING
320 Broad Street
Red Bank, NJ 07701

First originally published by Newman Springs Publishing 2020

ISBN 978-1-64801-223-5 (Paperback)
ISBN 978-1-64801-224-2 (Hardcover)
ISBN 978-1-64801-225-9 (Digital)

Printed in the United States of America

To all the families who have welcomed me into
their lives to help them help their children

The exercises in this book are not diagnostic for developmental concerns. If you have concerns about the development of your child, please consult with a developmental professional. Please make sure you feel comfortable doing these exercises with your child. If at any time you feel uncomfortable, please discontinue the exercises and contact a developmental or movement specialist. Never force your child into the position, especially if you feel it is painful for them. By doing these exercises, you take responsibility for your child's safety.

Contents

Why I Created Meaningful Moves

I have been asked more times than I can count, "What can I do to help my child's vision develop?" The answer to this question should be easy because, for most children, visual skills develop along with other sensory and motor skills without requiring intervention. But many of the parents I speak with are looking for guidance on how to do more for their child. I believe starting as early as possible is key.

The five Meaningful Moves exercises in this book stimulate sensory and motor skill development throughout the whole body. They are designed for babies, toddlers and young children who are developing well, and for those with developmental concerns. A baby's prenatal and birth experiences may impact the status of their nervous system. These exercises can help create balance in the body to allow for more optimal development. When a child knows where they are in space and knows how to move the body, vision is easily integrated into all daily tasks.

My hope is that Meaningful Moves helps prevent some of the developmental concerns that seem to be increasing among our children. I strive to educate and empower parents to be actively involved in their child's development. We don't need fancy strollers or apparatuses to contain our babies. We don't need an electronic device or new app to entertain them. Rather, we need to help our children move in meaningful ways to teach them where they are and how they can safely and efficiently interact with the things they see. Meaningful Moves can help.

Good luck,
Dr. Lane
XOXO

I Have Hands

It's with our hands that we touch. It's with our hands that we feel. We experience the world through using our hands to reach out to the things that we see. This Meaningful Move is designed to organize neurological circuits in the hands to provide a firm foundation for how we use our hands and how they help us gather information about our world.

This move can be done several times each day.

Here are the steps:

1. Starting at the base of the pointer finger, using firm pressure, smoothly move across the base of the fingers toward the base of the pinky finger. Repeat this motion three times.
2. After completing step 1, using the same pressure, move down the outside of the palm toward the heel of the hand. Repeat this motion three times.
3. After completing step 2, move across the heel of the hand, using the same firm pressure. Repeat this motion three times.
4. The last step is to move from the base of the thumb back up to the base of the pointer finger. Repeat this motion three times.
5. Repeat all steps on the other hand.

As you complete this motion you have provided stimulation to many nerves and reflexes that are responsible for how the hand moves and gathers information about the world.

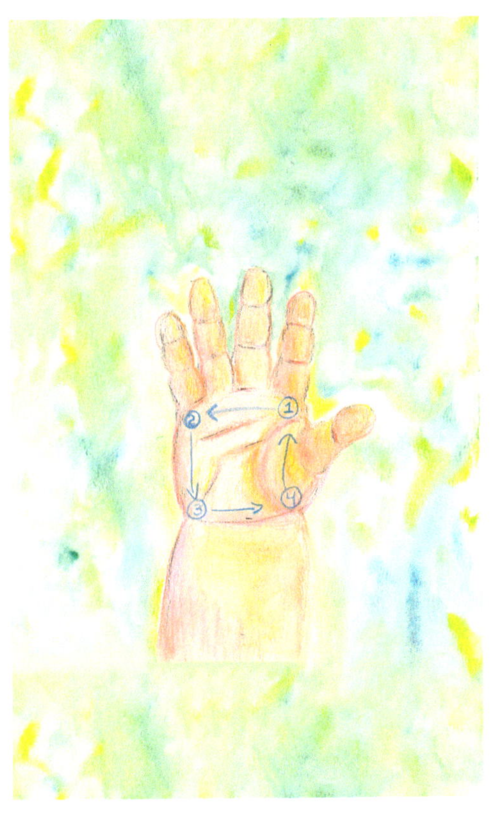

My HANDs can touch.
My HANDs can feel.
My HANDs can help me
move toward what I see.

I Have Feet

Our feet are our foundation. With every step we take we gather information about where we are and where we are going. When standing still, our feet help us to stay steady and grounded. When we are moving, our feet make the first move that guides our whole body. This Meaningful Move is designed to provide each foot with information about how to feel and move.

This move can be done several times a day.

Here are the steps:

1. On the bottom of the foot, use your thumb to apply pressure to the spot marked (1). Apply gentle pressure as you move smoothly up toward the base of the pinky toe.
2. After you complete step 1, stretch the big toe back, toward the knee. Hold for three seconds.
3. After you complete step 2, apply gentle pressure as you move down the arch of the foot.
4. Repeat steps 1–3 several times on each foot.

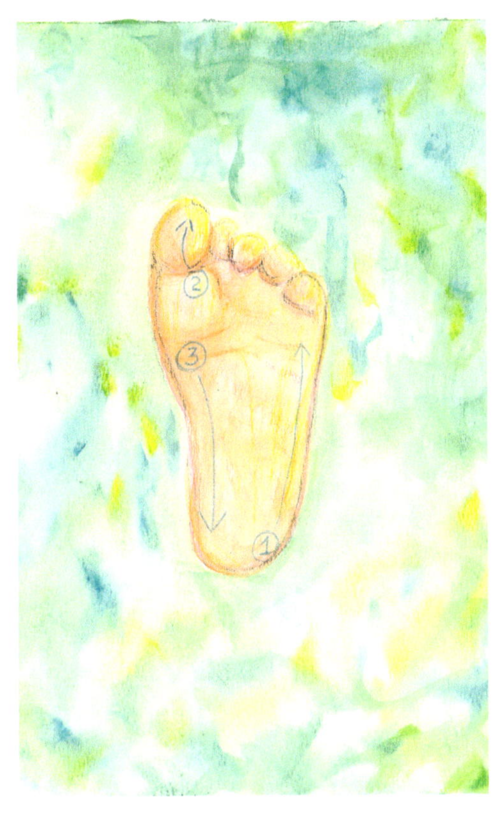

My FEET can move.
My FEET can feel.
My FEET help me know
where I am
and where I'm going.

I Can Go Side to Side

This Meaningful Move helps to discover movement through space. As we move side to side, we cross the middle of our bodies and switch from using the right side to using the left side. As our arms and legs move, our head follows.

The move is *slow* and rhythmical. Allow time for the information to be received.

Here are the steps while the child is lying on their back:

1. Gently grasp hands and feet together.
2. Slowly move the left foot across the body and bring it to touch the floor on the right side of the body. Pause. Allow time for the head to follow. You may notice that the forehead moves to touch the floor as full rotation of the head happens.
3. Slowly move back through the center position and move the right foot across the body to come to the floor on the left side of the body. Again, allow time for the head to follow.
4. Repeat this move for at least five cycles. Moving *slow* and *rhythmical.*

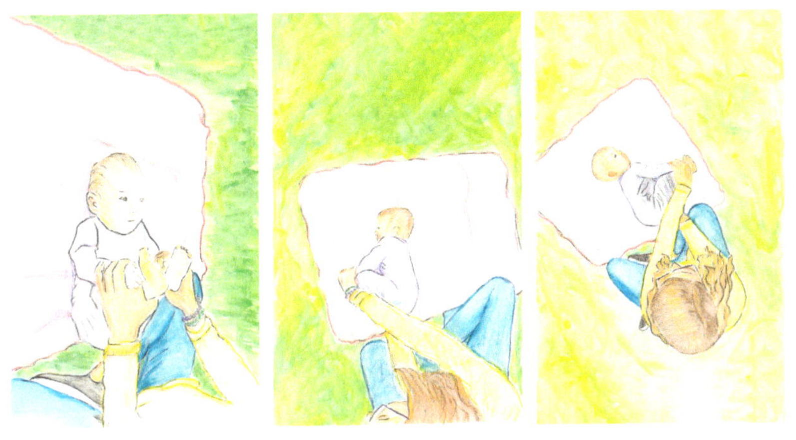

I can move to my RIGHT.
I can move to my LEFT.

My eyes and my head can follow
as my body moves from
SIDE to SIDE.

I Can Go Up and Down

This Meaningful Move works to stimulate all the nerves of the body. As we move up and down on the spine, we organize the flow of information throughout the entire body.

This move is *slow* and *rhythmical*. Allow time for the information to be received.

Here are the steps while the child is lying on their back:

1. Cup your hands under the bottom, with your finger tips resting at the top of the hip crest.
2. Gently begin to move up and then down.
3. Over time you can move to bring the feet to the forehead as you move up and then extend the legs out straight as you move down.
4. Repeat these steps up to ten times in one sitting.

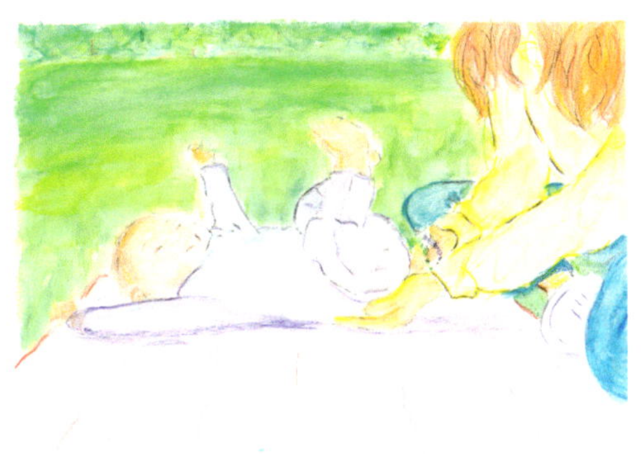

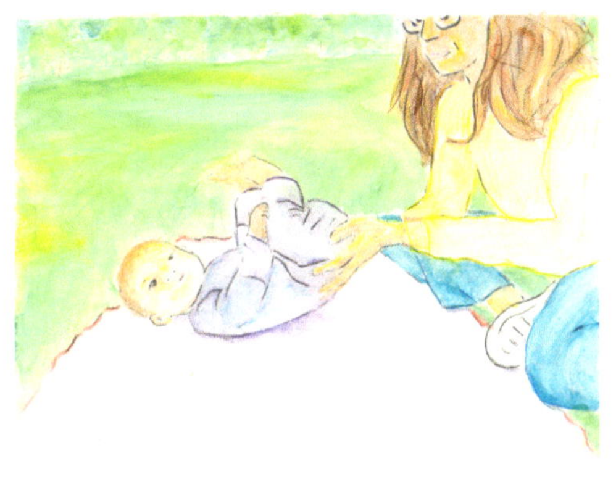

I

can

go

UP!

I can go DOWN!

My body can move smoothly

through space.

I Can Go Upside Down

This Meaningful Move helps to encourage the development of the reflexes needed for strong head and neck control as well as the reflexes needed to help protect you when you fall. This move can be scary at first but when practiced regularly becomes fun quickly.

Here are the steps:

1. With the child on his back facing toward you, firmly grasp around the hips. Your thumbs behind the back, at the top of the hip crest and your fingers across the lower belly and hips. Your grip must be steady and your strength enough to hold the child in the air safely. Please use caution when doing this exercise to make sure that you do not drop the child.

2. Slowly lift the hips up as the spine rolls along the floor.

3. Smoothly roll the baby and as the roll completes and the back of the head is the only part of the body still on the ground, lift the baby into the air.

4. Hold the baby in the air for a few moments, when you see the head move back, the back begin to arch and the arms extend toward the ground, gently place the baby back down with the hands being the first part of the body to touch the ground, followed by the belly and then the knees.

5. This exercise can be repeated several times. If you do not see the head move back, the back arch, or the hands extend, repeat the motion but while holding the child in the air, bring him toward the ground but not touching it. Repeat this 3–5 times and watch for development of the movements. If you still do not see the movements, bring the child down gently with the head touching, then the chest, and then the whole body. Continue with this exercise even if you don't see the expected response, it will come with time.

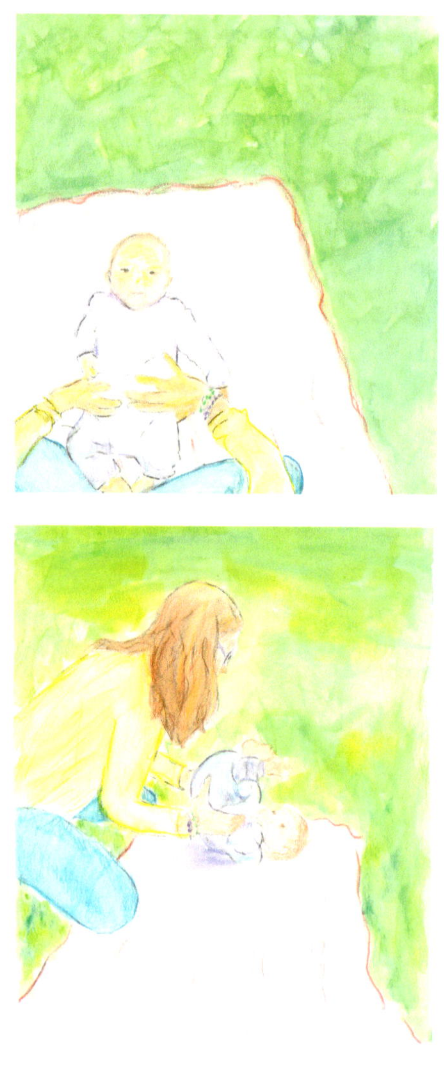

Hold me steady. Hold me strong.

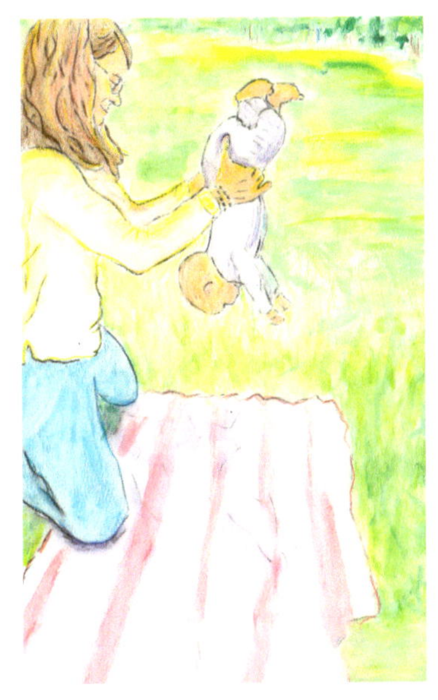

I can flip upside down.

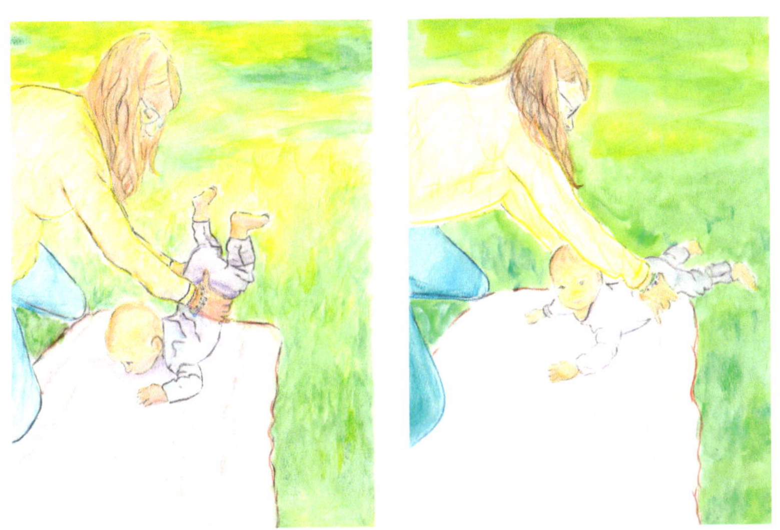

About the Illustrator

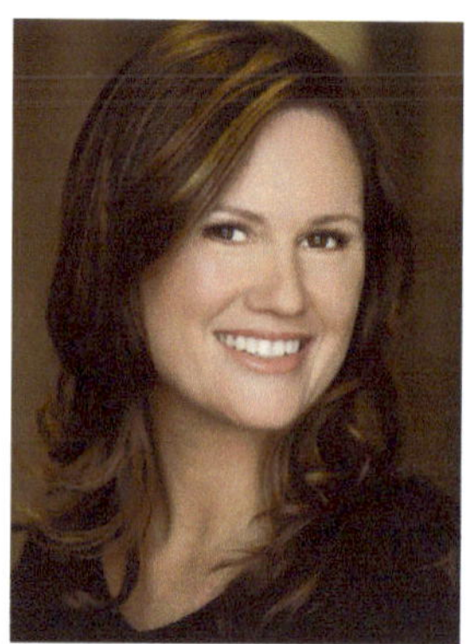

Elizabeth Barker is an artist, an actress, and a teacher of art. Being a lifelong resident of the Jersey Shore, she draws her inspiration from local beaches as well as nearby New York City. Her work is predominantly executed in acrylic paint on canvas. Visit her at elizabethbarker.net and on Instagram @_elizabethbarker.

About the Author

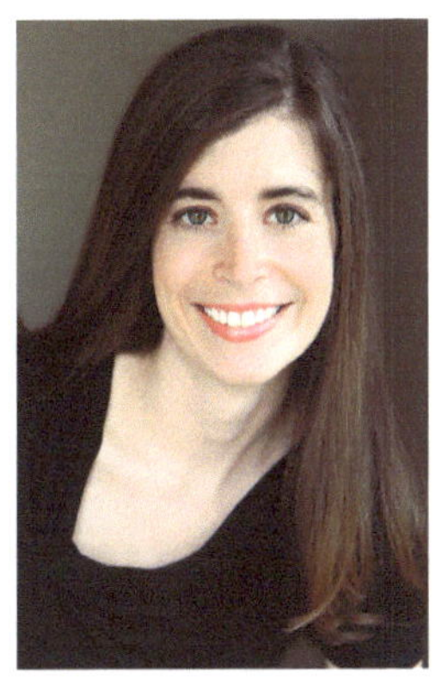

Dr. Lane is a developmental optometrist, a specialized eye doctor who is concerned more with how a person uses what they see than if a they have perfect eyesight. After integrating yoga practice into her own vision therapy, Dr. Lane became passionate about the connection between the whole body and the visual process. Her appreciation for the importance of an organized body intensified when she became a parent, and watched as her own children developed the skills needed to safely navigate their world.

In 2010, Dr. Lane cofounded Natural Beginnings: Resources for Growing Families, a community center that integrated her interests in holistic lifestyle with her love of developmental optometry. She developed Meaningful Moves to empower parents to provide home based opportunities for sensorimotor development from birth through childhood. Currently, Dr. Lane sees patients at the FOCUS Center for Vision and Learning, in New Jersey.

After graduating from Pennsylvania College of Optometry, Dr. Lane completed residency at SUNY Optometry in 2006. She is a certified yoga teacher, a HypnoBirthing Childbirth Educator, and a student of many body movement and reflex integration methods.